Liver Diet Cookbook For Beginners

The Easy Guide To Maintain Your Liver Health Routine And To Cook Tasty Recipes In The Best Way Possible

Loren Allen

© Copyright 2021 by Loren Allen - All rights reserved.

The following Book is reproduced below with the goal of providing information that is as accurate and reliable as possible. Regardless, purchasing this Book can be seen as consent to the fact that both the publisher and the author of this book are in no way experts on the topics discussed within and that any recommendations or suggestions that are made herein are for entertainment purposes only. Professionals should be consulted as needed prior to undertaking any of the action endorsed herein.

This declaration is deemed fair and valid by both the American Bar Association and the Committee of Publishers Association and is legally binding throughout the United States.

Furthermore, the transmission, duplication, or reproduction of any of the following work including specific information will be considered an illegal act irrespective of if it is done electronically or in print. This extends to creating a secondary or tertiary copy of the work or a recorded copy and is only allowed with the express written consent from the Publisher. All additional right reserved.

The information in the following pages is broadly considered a truthful and accurate account of facts and as such, any inattention, use, or misuse of the information in question by the reader will render any resulting actions solely under their purview. There are no scenarios in which the publisher or the original author of this work can be in any fashion deemed liable for any hardship or damages that may befall them after undertaking information described herein.

Additionally, the information in the following pages is intended only for informational purposes and should thus be thought of as universal. As befitting its nature, it is presented without assurance regarding its prolonged validity or interim quality. Trademarks that are mentioned are done without written consent and can in no way be considered an endorsement from the trademark holder.

Table Of Contents

Your Liver is a true superhero! — 8

Cirrhosis: How Healthy Are Your Livers? — 10

Functions Of The Liver - The Liver: Your Body's Most Important Muscle — 17

Discovering the Stages of Liver Failure — 23

    Liver failure vs. liver disease — 25

    Stages of liver failure — 26

    Causes of liver failure — 28

    Symptoms of acute liver failure — 31

    Symptoms of chronic liver failure — 31

    Diagnosing liver failure — 33

    What are the treatment options for liver failure? — 35

    Preventing liver failure — 37

    Outlook — 38

    Cucumber-basil Salsa On Halibut Pouches — 39

    Light & Creamy Garlic Hummus — 42

Polenta Cups Recipe	44
Roasted Asparagus	46
Seafood Stew Cioppino	47
Veggie Balls	49
Cod With Lentils	51
Stuffed Mackerel	53
Collard Greens And Tomatoes	55
Sage Salmon Fillet	56
Baked Sweet-potato Fries	57
Scallions Dip	60
Blueberry Granola Bars	61
Chicken Kale Wraps	63
Vinegar Beet Bites	65
Strawberry Frozen Yogurt	66
Tasty Black Bean Dip	68
Homemade Nutella	70
Oatmeal Cookies	71
Chili-lime Cucumber, Jicama, & Apple Sticks	73

Sardine Meatballs	74
Homemade Salsa	76
Kale Chips	78
Feta Tomato Sea Bass	79
Crab Stew	81
Trail Mix	83
Berry & Veggie Gazpacho	84
Meat-filled Phyllo (samboosek)	85
Raw Turmeric Cashew Nut & Coconut Balls	87
Ginger Tahini Dip With Veggies	89
Crunchy Veggie Chips	90
Honey Garlic Shrimp	91
Pita Chips	93
Leeks And Calamari Mix	95
Cucumber Rolls	96
Parmesan Chips	97
Grape, Celery & Parsley Reviver	99
Tomato Triangles	100

Asparagus Frittata	101
Salmon And Broccoli	103
Chili Mango And Watermelon Salsa	104
Chia Crackers	105
Lavash Roll Ups	107
Pepper Salmon Skewers	109
Garlic Mussels	111
Superfood Spiced Apricot-sesame Bliss Balls	113
Halibut And Quinoa Mix	115
Orange-spiced Pumpkin Hummus	117
Artichoke Skewers	118
Honey Balsamic Salmon	119
Conclusion	**121**

Your Liver is a true superhero!

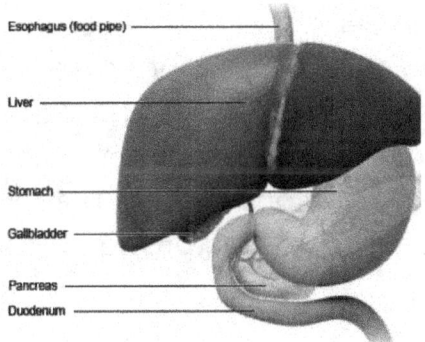

The liver is an essential organ that helps us digest food, process toxins and metabolize nutrients. If damage from cirrhosis means the function of your liver isn't as efficient anymore, a specific diet might be able to provide you with all necessary nutritional support without pushing it too hard.

Research has shown that people who are suffering from hepatic diseases like hepatitis or cirrhosis are at risk for complications such as death if they don't receive enough nourishment (emphasis on protein) through their diets; so be sure not to skip meals!

A 2018 article in the Journal of Clinical Gastroenterology states that "dietary management should be implemented earlier on to improve clinical prognosis."

If you have liver cirrhosis, then it's important to stay on top of your diet. If not managed well enough, scarring will continue and worsen which can lead to a number of issues such as an increased risk for cancer or bleeding due to the organ being unable provide blood clotting capability.

If you're concerned about whether managing your diet is something that would be too much trouble for someone with hepatic impairment; don't worry - there are plenty of recipes out there available at any grocery store in most major cities! There should also be information readily available online if one need help finding their way through cooking healthy dishes easily without sacrificing taste.

Cirrhosis: How Healthy Are Your Livers?

The Mediterranean Diet and a few supplements like milk thistle can help limit weight loss while limiting progression of liver disease.

You want to avoid high-sugar beverages as well because they are very hard for your body's immune system when it is fighting an infection or just recovering from one!

In short, remember, eat food that is soft, avoid drinking alcohol, don't eat foods that are spicy.

1. Nutrition in Early Liver Cirrhosis Disease

Food

A healthy diet should consist of a variety of foods high in nutrients and vitamins. Healthy choices include fruit, vegetables, whole grains, lean protein sources such as chicken breast or tofu, unsalted nuts and seeds like walnuts or almonds for some crunchy texture to your meal on the side. Dairy products provide calcium needed for strong bones but be sure not to add too much fat with milk cheeses because they are higher in saturated fats than low-fat dairy options without cheese that will help keep you full longer after eating them - perfect before bedtime snacks! Keep sodium content lower by avoiding ketchup which is surprisingly one food containing large amounts of salt per serving size at 560mg/1 tbsp., pickles also contain an average 77% more

Selecting foods with healthy fats is important. Choosing unsaturated fats instead of saturated fats and trans fats is a good first step. Unsaturated fats:

- include monosaturated, polyunsaturated and Omega3 fatty acids

- come from plant sources and fish and include avocado, nuts, olive oil, canola oil and safflower oil

- foods high in Omega3 fatty acids include salmon, tuna and mackerel

Beverages

Drink water. Drinking too much sugar is bad for your body and may lead to weight gain or diabetes. Keep in mind that coffee can be good for you, but only up to three cups each day - any more than this could cause a variety of health problems including liver disease like cirrhosis! As always, it's important not to drink alcohol when the goal is improved liver health.

Vitamins and Minerals

Vitamins are the best way to keep you healthy, even if that's all you're eating is a variety of unhealthy foods. One exception would be in cases where someone has alcoholic liver disease and thiamine (vitamin B1), folic acid, and multivitamins should be taken- this includes vitamins B2 and B6 as well. If your diagnosis doesn't include hemochromatosis then vitamin C can also help prevent illness which may arise from an imbalance between iron absorption or retention levels due to genetics or autoimmune conditions such as celiac disease .

Vitamins provide much needed nutrients for many people who might not otherwise get them through their diet alone! An example would be those with alcohol related liver diseases; they

2. Nutrition in Advanced Liver Cirrhosis Disease

Food

Poor appetite, nausea and vomiting can lead to malnutrition in advanced liver disease (ALD). Loss of protein from decreased absorption or increased losses also contribute. Protein is not restricted even with ALD but you should avoid large amounts due the fact that your body does not store it well. Eating small meals more frequently may be better tolerated by an individual with ALD since they are much easier for their now-defunct liver to process than larger ones would be at one sitting time per day--this will also help keep them feeling full longer!

ALD causes the kidneys to hold sodium (salt) which then results in your body holding more fluid thus increasing ascites (swollen abdomen) and swelling of the hands, legs and feet. Your provider may ask that you restrict your sodium intake to 2000 mg or less (1 teaspoon of salt contains approximately 2300mg sodium). Sodium in all foods and beverages must be calculated into this amount. Reading sodium content on packaging will be necessary. You should remember that the sodium content on the package is for the serving size indicated on the label, not for the entire amount of the package. If you have chronic kidney disease, salt substitutes should be avoided because they are high in potassium.

Beverages

Your provider will tell you if or when to restrict your fluid intake with liver disease. The goal is 1500-2000 ml per day, but more than that can be prescribed by a doctor in order alleviate symptoms of feeling thirsty which could stem from taking diuretics (water pills). One way to keep track of how much water you drink for the whole day would be filling up one pitcher and every time we drink something take out an equivalent amount of water so it never goes below this limit! If on a restricted diet due to being on these medications, there are tricks such as drinking soup instead because they still count towards the daily total. Sugar-free frozen pops, sugar-free sour candy, sugar-free gelatin, sucking on lemon or lime slices and eating ice cold fruit and vegetables will help relieve thirst. Frozen grapes are a good option. Fluid from the sugar-free frozen pops and gelatin must be included in the daily allowance of fluid intake, as will the fluid in juicy fruit like watermelon.

Vitamins and Minerals

There is a fine line between not enough and too much when taking vitamin supplements. When you are sick, it may be difficult to know what the right amount of vitamins for your illness might be if you aren't sure of their effects on an already broken system. For example, excessive amounts can injure your liver which is at risk in this case because they have also been depleted from other illnesses such as Jaundice (yellow skin and eyes).

Fatigue, muscle weakness and twitches and cramps of your arms, hands and feet may indicate magnesium deficiency in ALD. Your provider may order a blood test to determine magnesium level and, if low, a supplement will be ordered. ALD may also cause a zinc deficiency. Signs of a zinc deficiency include decreased appetite, decreased ability to fight infection, diarrhea and hair loss. A zinc supplement may be ordered by your provider. Muscle cramps can also be relieved with drinking either regular or diet tonic water because of the quinine content. It is important not to drink more than 4 ounces per day because of the high sodium content.

Functions Of The Liver - The Liver: Your Body's Most Important Muscle

The liver is the largest organ in your body and without it life would be impossible. The liver's job includes filtering blood, maintaining healthy sugar levels, regulating clotting of blood (which prevents you from bleeding excessively), and performing hundreds more tasks that keep us alive. Located just under our ribs on the right side of our abdomen, this most important muscle helps fight infection by making new cells to replace dying ones!

Key Facts

The liver filters all of the blood in the body and breaks down poisonous substances, such as alcohol and drugs.

The liver also produces bile, a fluid that helps digest fats and carry away waste.

The liver consists of four lobes, which are each made up of eight sections and thousands of lobules (or small lobes).

Functions of the Liver

The liver is the body's trash compactor, producing essential blood sugars and nutrients. It also removes waste products from your bloodstream to provide you with a squeaky-clean circulatory system!

A lot of people might not be aware that their liver does so much work for them every day, but it really can't do everything without some help or support either - just like any other muscle in your body needs extra care when tired after working out. That said, there are healthy diet options to give yourself an energy boost so that this important organ doesn't have as tough a time performing its functions throughout the course of our 24 hour lifespan.

Albumin Production: Albumin is a protein that keeps fluids in the bloodstream from leaking into surrounding tissue. It also carries hormones, vitamins, and enzymes through the body.

Bile Production: Bile is a fluid that is critical to the digestion and absorption of fats in the small intestine.

Filters Blood: All the blood leaving the stomach and intestines passes through the liver, which removes toxins, byproducts, and other harmful substances.

Regulates Amino Acids: The production of proteins depend on amino acids. The liver makes sure amino acid levels in the bloodstream remain healthy.

Regulates Blood Clotting: Blood clotting coagulants are created using vitamin K, which can only be absorbed with the help of bile, a fluid the liver produces.

Resists Infections: As part of the filtering process, the liver also removes bacteria from the bloodstream.

Stores Vitamins and Minerals: The liver stores significant amounts of vitamins A, D, E, K, and B12, as well as iron and copper.

Processes Glucose: The liver removes excess glucose (sugar) from the bloodstream and stores it as glycogen. As needed, it can convert glycogen back into glucose.

Anatomy of the Liver

The liver is reddish-brown and shaped approximately like a cone or a wedge, with the small end above the spleen and stomach and the large end above the small intestine. The entire organ is located below the lungs in the right upper abdomen. It weighs between 3 and 3.5 pounds.

Structure

The liver is a large organ that consists of four lobes. The two larger, right lobe and left lobe are divided by the falciform ligament, which connects the liver to the abdominal wall. These segments can be further subdivided into eight smaller ones each with its own ducts for bile (a digestive fluid).

Parts

The following are some of the most important individual parts of the liver:

Common Hepatic Duct: A tube that carries bile out of the liver. It is formed from the intersection of the right and left hepatic ducts.

Falciform Ligament: A thin, fibrous ligament that separates the two lobes of the liver and connects it to the abdominal wall.

Glisson's Capsule: A layer of loose connective tissue that surrounds the liver and its related arteries and ducts.

Hepatic Artery: The main blood vessel that supplies the liver with oxygenated blood.

Hepatic Portal Vein: The blood vessel that carries blood from the gastrointestinal tract, gallbladder, pancreas, and spleen to the liver.

Lobes: The anatomical sections of the liver.

Lobules: Microscopic building blocks of the liver.

Peritoneum: A membrane covering the liver that forms the exterior.

Maintaining a Healthy Liver

The best way to avoid liver disease is by taking active steps towards a healthy life. The following are some recommendations that will help keep the liver functioning as it should:

Avoid Illicit Drugs: Illicit drugs are toxins that the liver must filter out. Taking these drugs can cause long-term damage.

Drink Alcohol Moderately: Alcohol must be broken down by the liver. While the liver can moderate amounts, excessive alcohol use can cause damage.

Exercise Regularly: A regular exercise routine will help promote general health for every organ, including the liver.

Eat Healthy Foods: Eating excessive fats can make it difficult for the liver to function and lead to fatty liver disease.

Practice Safe Sex: Use protection to avoid sexually transmitted diseases such as hepatitis C.

Vaccinate: Especially when traveling, get appropriate vaccinations against hepatitis A and B, as well as diseases such as malaria and yellow fever, which grow in the liver.

Discovering the Stages of Liver Failure

Liver failure is a life-threatening emergency. The two main types of liver failures are acute or chronic and it can either come on quickly, like when one has an infection that leads to increased alcohol abuse or if you're born with certain genetics (such as hemochromatosis), whereas the other type occurs gradually over time in some people who may not have any risks factors for developing their disease but just develop them due to lifestyle choices.

Acute liver failure suddenly comes on while chronic cases happen slowly over weeks/months so they're easier treated before serious damage happens; however, this doesn't mean your symptoms will go away because there's no cure--only treatments--and many sufferers don't know about early signs which could be monitored.

The liver is an important part of the body. It can be damaged and not work properly. The damage can happen in stages that get worse over time.

Stages of liver failure

Inflammation. In this early stage, the liver is enlarged or inflamed.

Fibrosis. Scar tissue begins to replace healthy tissue in the inflamed liver.

Cirrhosis. Severe scarring has built up, making it difficult for the liver to function properly.

End-stage liver disease (ESLD). Liver function has deteriorated to the point where the damage can't be reversed other than with a liver transplant.

Liver cancer. The development and multiplication of unhealthy cells in the liver can occur at any stage of liver failure, although people with cirrhosis are more at risk.

Liver failure vs. liver disease

The liver is one of the most important organs in your body. There are many different types of diseases that can affect it, but two specific ones to watch out for are degenerative and acute hepatitis. The first usually causes damage over time while the latter often occurs quickly due to rapid infection or injury from an outside source like alcohol abuse or a car accident. These conditions result in inflammation, pain, swelling and even death if left untreated! It's good you know what these look like so when they come up on your medical tests you'll be able to react appropriately instead of waiting around until something more serious happens again later down the line.

Stages of liver failure

Damage from liver disease can happen in stages. The damage goes up and it makes the liver not work as well.

Inflammation

In this early stage, your liver becomes swollen or inflamed. Many people with this condition do not have symptoms. If it continues for a long time, your liver can be permanently damaged.

Fibrosis

Fibrosis is inflammation of the liver. This can happen when the liver starts to scar.

The scar tissue that's generated in this stage replaces healthy liver tissue. But the scarred tissue can't do what the healthy tissue did. It can start to affect your liver's ability to work right.

Fibrosis is hard to notice because there are not usually any symptoms.

Cirrhosis

When you have cirrhosis, your liver is damaged. That means it doesn't work as well.

When you first get liver disease, you may not have any symptoms. But now, you might start to feel bad.

End-stage liver disease (ESLD)

People with ESLD have a disease called cirrhosis. This means that the liver has been damaged.

ESLD is associated with complications such as ascites and hepatic encephalopathy. It can't be reversed unless you get a liver transplant.

Liver cancer

Cancer is when cells in your body are not healthy. If you have cancer in your liver, it is called primary liver cancer.

Although it can happen at any stage of liver failure, people with cirrhosis are more likely to get liver cancer.

Some common symptoms of liver cancer include:

- unexplained weight loss
- abdominal pain or swelling
- loss of appetite or feeling full after eating a small amount of food
- nausea or vomiting
- yellowing of the skin and eyes (jaundice)
- skin itching

Causes of liver failure

The cause of liver failure can depend on the type of liver failure — acute or chronic.

Causes of acute liver failure

Acute liver failure occurs quickly. It can be caused by many things, but sometimes the exact cause is unknown.. Some possible causes include:

- A viral infection happens when a virus enters the body. There are three viruses that can cause infections: hepatitis A, B, or E.
- A person might overdose on acetaminophen (Tylenol) if they take too much.
- There are many different reactions to prescription medicines. For example, some people might have a reaction when they use antibiotics, NSAIDs or anti-epileptic drugs.
- Reactions to herbal supplements, such as ma huang and kava kava.
- metabolic conditions, such as Wilson's disease
- autoimmune conditions are when your body attacks itself. For example, there is autoimmune hepatitis.
- If you have the condition where the veins of your liver are affected, like Budd-Chiari syndrome, then it is important to eat less fat.
- Exposure to toxins can happen in the workplace or when you eat a bad mushroom.

Causes of chronic liver failure

Liver failure happens when a person's liver gets hurt over time. This can lead to cirrhosis, which is when there is too much scar tissue on the liver and it stops working right.

Some examples of possible causes of cirrhosis include:

- chronic hepatitis B or C infection
- Alcohol-related liver disease (ARLD) is a disease that can happen when you drink alcohol. It happens in your liver.
- Nonalcoholic fatty liver disease means that someone has a lot of fat in their liver and they do not drink alcohol.
- autoimmune hepatitis
- Diseases that affect your bile duct can be very bad. They are called cholangitis.

Symptoms of acute liver failure

Acute liver failure can happen to people who do not have a condition in their liver. This is an emergency and people should see a doctor when they have symptoms that are like acute liver failure.

The symptoms of acute liver failure can include:

- feeling unwell (malaise)
- feeling tired or sleepy
- nausea or vomiting
- abdominal pain or swelling
- yellowing of the skin and eyes (jaundice)
- feeling confused or disoriented

Symptoms of chronic liver failure

Some symptoms of chronic liver failure are early symptoms and some are more advanced. Early symptoms may include:

- feeling tired or fatigued
- loss of appetite
- nausea or vomiting
- mild abdominal discomfort or pain

Some symptoms that might mean you have a liver problem are:

- yellowing of the skin and eyes (jaundice)
- easy bruising or bleeding
- feeling confused or disoriented
- buildup of fluid in your abdomen, arms, or legs
- darkening of your urine
- severe skin itching

Diagnosing liver failure

To diagnose liver failure, your doctor will start by taking your medical history and performing a physical examination. They may then perform additional tests to rule out other causes of symptoms such as: blood work-up for anemia or anaemia; chest X-ray to look at the lungs and heart health; EKG for an irregular heartbeat (arrhythmia); urinalysis looking at kidney function along with electrolytes in urine samples.; imaging scans like ultrasounds or CTs which can visualize different parts of our body.

You might also have some generalized pain around the abdomen area that you'll need to mention on this list too!

- A **liver blood test** is a test to see how your liver is working. There are different proteins and enzymes in the blood, and these can tell.
- **Other blood tests.** Your doctor can do a blood test to see if you have any problems in your liver. There are many different tests that they can do.
- **Imaging tests.** Ultrasound, CT scan, and MRI can help your doctor to see your liver.
- **Biopsy.** Taking a tissue sample of your liver can help your doctor see if there is scar tissue or other reasons for your condition.

What are the treatment options for liver failure?

The liver is important for our body. We need it to help us do things like digest food, and if it doesn't work, then we will have a problem. If there is something going wrong with our liver, then we might have to take medicine or get surgery so that the damage can stop happening.

For example, antiviral medications can be used to treat a viral hepatitis infection, or immune suppressing medication can be given to treat autoimmune hepatitis.

Lifestyle changes may also be recommended as a part of your treatment. These can include things like abstaining from alcohol, losing weight, or avoiding the use of certain medications.

The American Liver Foundation estimates that a large percentage of the damage to your liver can be reversed, if caught and treated. If not, this may lead to cirrhosis or ESLD which is often irreversible but sometimes slows down progression.

What about acute liver failure?

Acute liver failure is often treated in the intensive care unit of a hospital. Supportive care can be given to help stabilize your condition and control any complications during treatment and recovery from acute liver failure.

A medication overdose or reaction may also lead you to receive drugs that reverse its effects, while a potential indication for transplantation may exist for some people with this type of serious medical emergency due to their severe illness severity, which could even progress into coma if left untreated too long!

Preventing liver failure

You can help to prevent liver failure by making lifestyle changes. If you make them, your liver will be happy and healthy. Here are some tips for improving liver health:

- Drink alcohol in moderation, and never mix medications with alcohol.
- Take medications only when needed, and carefully follow any dosing instructions.
- Don't mix medications without first consulting your doctor.
- To maintain a healthy weight, there is a connection to liver disease.
- Get vaccinated against hepatitis A and B.
- Be sure to have regular physicals with your doctor during which they perform liver blood tests.

Outlook

Liver failure is when your liver can't function properly. It can be either acute or chronic, and in the later stages of life it may require a transplant to save lives. Liver deterioration could have been caused by alcoholism, hepatitis-C infection, cancer treatment side effects such as chemotherapy drugs that damage the healthy cells along with tumor cells; or even radiation for kidney stones where some parts of belly will get more exposed than others due to increased urination which was previously being handled by kidneys before they were damaged from stone disease - you name it! In any case though whether its just one factor like alcohol abuse leading up to cirrhosis and then eventually hepatocellular carcinoma (liver cancer) if untreated through surgery followed.

People who are diagnosed with liver disease are often monitored throughout their life to make sure that their condition isn't worsening or causing further liver damage. If you have concerns about liver health or about liver failure, be sure to talk to your doctor.

Cucumber-basil Salsa On Halibut Pouches

Servings: 3

Cooking Time: 17 Minutes

Ingredients:

- 1 lime, thinly sliced into 8 pieces
- 2 cups mustard greens, stems removed
- 2 tsp olive oil
- 4 – 5 radishes trimmed and quartered
- 4 4-oz skinless halibut filets
- 4 large fresh basil leaves
- Cayenne pepper to taste – optional
- Pepper and salt to taste
- 1 ½ cups diced cucumber
- 1 ½ finely chopped fresh basil leaves
- 2 tsp fresh lime juice
- Pepper and salt to taste

Directions:

1. Preheat oven to 400oF.
2. Preparation are parchment papers by making 4 pieces of 15 x 12-inch rectangles. Lengthwise, fold in half and unfold pieces on the table.
3. Season halibut fillets with pepper, salt and cayenne—if using cayenne.
4. Just to the right of the fold going lengthwise, place ½ cup of mustard greens. Add a basil leaf on center of mustard greens and topped with 1 lime slice. Around the greens, layer ¼ of the radishes. Drizzle with ½ tsp of oil, season with pepper and salt. Top it with a slice of halibut fillet.
5. Just as you would make a calzone, fold parchment paper over your filling and crimp the edges of the parchment paper beginning from one end to the other end. To seal the end of the crimped parchment paper, pinch it.
6. Repeat process to remaining ingredients until you have 4 pieces of parchment papers filled with halibut and greens.
7. Place pouches in a baking pan and bake in the oven until halibut is flaky, around 15 to 17 minutes.

8. While waiting for halibut pouches to cook, make your salsa by mixing all salsa ingredients in a medium bowl.
9. Once halibut is cooked, remove from oven and make a tear on top. Be careful of the steam as it is very hot. Equally divide salsa and spoon ¼ of salsa on top of halibut through the slit you have created.
10. Serve and enjoy

Nutrition:

Calories per serving: 335.4; Protein: 20.2g; Fat: 16.3g; Carbs: 22.1g

Light & Creamy Garlic Hummus

Servings: 10

Cooking Time: 40 Minutes

Ingredients:

- 1 1/2 cups dry chickpeas, rinsed
- 2 1/2 tbsp fresh lemon juice
- 1 tbsp garlic, minced
- 1/2 cup tahini
- 6 cups of water
- Pepper
- Salt

Directions:

- Add water and chickpeas into the instant pot.
- Seal pot with a lid and select manual and set timer for 40 minutes.
- Once done, allow to release pressure naturally. Remove lid.
- Drain chickpeas well and reserved 1/2 cup chickpeas liquid.
- Transfer chickpeas, reserved liquid, lemon juice, garlic, tahini, pepper, and salt into the food processor and process until smooth.
- Serve and enjoy

Nutrition:

Calories 152 Fat 6.9 g Carbohydrates 17.6 g Sugar 2.8 g Protein 6.6 g Cholesterol 0 mg

Polenta Cups Recipe

Servings:3

Cooking Time:20 Minutes

Ingredients:

- 1 cup yellow cornmeal
- 1 garlic clove, minced
- 1/2 teaspoon fresh thyme, minced or 1/4 teaspoon dried thyme
- 1/2 teaspoon salt
- 1/4 cup feta cheese, crumbled
- 1/4 teaspoon pepper
- 2 tablespoons fresh basil, chopped
- 4 cups water
- 4 plum tomatoes, finely chopped

Directions:

- In a heavy, large saucepan, bring the water and the salt to a boil; reduce the heat to a gentle boil. Slowly whisk in the cornmeal; cook, stirring with a wooden spoon for about 15 to 20 minutes, or until the polenta is thick and pulls away cleanly from the sides of the pan. Remove from the heat; stir in the pepper and the thyme.
- Grease miniature muffin cups with cooking spray. Spoon a heaping tablespoon of the polenta mixture into each muffin cups.
- With the back of a spoon, make an indentation in the center of each; cover and chill until the mixture is set.
- Meanwhile, combine the feta cheese, tomatoes, garlic, and basil in a small-sized bowl.
- Unmold the chilled polenta cups; place them on an ungreased baking sheet. Tops each indentation with 1 heaping tablespoon of the feta mixture. Broil the cups 4 inches from the heat source for about 5 to 7 minutes, or until heated through.

Nutrition:

26 cal, 1 mg chol., 62 mg sodium, 5 g carbs., 1 g fiber, and 1 g protein.

Roasted Asparagus

Servings:3

Cooking Time:10 Minutes

Ingredients:

- 1 asparagus bunch, trimmed
- 3 tsp. avocado oil
- A splash of lemon juice
- Salt and ground black pepper to taste
- 1 tbsp. fresh oregano, chopped

Directions:

- Spread the asparagus spears on a lined baking sheet, season with salt, and pepper, drizzle with oil and lemon juice, sprinkle with oregano, and toss to coat well.
- Put in an oven at 425°F, and bake for 10 minutes.
- Divide onto plates and serve.

Nutrition:

Calories 130 ,Fat 1 g ,Carbs 2 g ,Protein 3 g

Seafood Stew Cioppino

Servings: 6

Cooking Time: 40 Minutes

Ingredients:

- ¼ cup Italian parsley, chopped
- ¼ tsp dried basil
- ¼ tsp dried thyme
- ½ cup dry white wine like pinot grigio
- ½ lb. King crab legs, cut at each joint
- ½ onion, chopped
- ½ tsp red pepper flakes (adjust to desired spiciness)
- 1 28-oz can crushed tomatoes
- 1 lb. mahi mahi, cut into ½-inch cubes
- 1 lb. raw shrimp
- 1 tbsp olive oil
- 2 bay leaves
- 2 cups clam juice
- 50 live clams, washed
- 6 cloves garlic, minced
- Pepper and salt to taste

Directions:

- On medium fire, place a stockpot and heat oil.
- Add onion and for 4 minutes sauté until soft.
- Add bay leaves, thyme, basil, red pepper flakes and garlic. Cook for a minute while stirring a bit.
- Add clam juice and tomatoes. Once simmering, place fire to medium low and cook for 20 minutes uncovered.
- Add white wine and clams. Cover and cook for 5 minutes or until clams have slightly opened.
- Stir pot then add fish pieces, crab legs and shrimps. Do not stir soup to maintain the fish's shape. Cook while covered for 4 minutes or until clams are fully opened; fish and shrimps are opaque and cooked.
- Season with pepper and salt to taste.
- Transfer Cioppino to serving bowls and garnish with parsley before serving.

Nutrition:

Calories per Serving: 371; Carbs: 15.5 g; Protein: 62 g; Fat: 6.8 g

Veggie Balls

Servings:3

Cooking Time:30 Minutes

Ingredients:

- 2 medium sweet potatoes, peeled and cubed into ½-inch size
- 2 tbsp. unsweetened coconut milk
- 1 C. fresh kale leaves, trimmed and chopped
- 1 medium shallot, chopped finely
- 1 tsp. ground cumin
- ½ tsp. granulated garlic
- ¼ tsp. ground turmeric
- Salt and freshly ground black pepper, to taste
- Ground flax seeds, as require

Directions:

- Preheat the oven to 400 degrees F. Line a baking sheet with parchment paper.
- In a pan of water, arrange a steamer basket.
- Place the sweet potato in steamer basket and steam for about 10-15 minutes.
- In a large bowl, place the sweet potato with the coconut milk and mash well.
- Add remaining ingredients except flax seeds and mix till well combined.
- Make about 1½-2-inch balls from the mixture.
- Arrange the balls onto preparation ared baking sheet in a single layer and sprinkle with flax seeds.
- Bake for about 20-25 minutes.

Nutrition:

448 Calories 27g fat 41g carbs 15g protein

Cod With Lentils

Servings:4

Cooking Time:30 Minutes

Ingredients:

- 1 red pepper, chopped
- 1 yellow onion, diced
- 1 teaspoon ground black pepper
- 1 teaspoon butter
- 1 jalapeno pepper, chopped
- ½ cup lentils
- 3 cups chicken stock
- 1 teaspoon salt
- 1 tablespoon tomato paste
- 1 teaspoon chili pepper
- 3 tablespoons fresh cilantro, chopped
- 8 oz cod, chopped

Directions:

- Place butter, red pepper, onion, and ground black pepper in the saucepan.
- Roast the vegetables for 5 minutes over the medium heat.
- Then add chopped jalapeno pepper, lentils, and chili pepper.
- Mix up the mixture well and add chicken stock and tomato paste.
- Stir until homogenous. Add cod.
- Close the lid and cook chili for 20 minutes over the medium heat

Nutrition:

calories 187, fat 2.3, fiber 8.8, carbs 21.3, protein 20.6

Stuffed Mackerel

Servings: 5

Cooking Time: 30 Minutes

Ingredients:

- 4 teaspoons capers, drained
- 1-pound whole mackerel, peeled, trimmed
- 1 teaspoon garlic powder
- ½ teaspoon ground coriander
- ½ teaspoon salt
- 1 tablespoon lime juice
- ¼ teaspoon chili flakes
- ½ white onion, sliced
- 4 teaspoons butter
- 3 tablespoons water

Directions:

- Rub the fish with salt, garlic powder, and chili flakes.
- Then sprinkle it with lime juice.
- Line the baking tray with parchment and arrange the fish inside.
- Fill the mackerel with capers and butter.
- Then sprinkle fish with water.
- Cover the fish with foil and secure the edges.
- Bake the mackerel for 30 minutes at 365F.

Nutrition:

calories 262, fat 17.5, fiber 0.4, carbs 1.8, protein 25.5

Collard Greens And Tomatoes

Servings:3

Cooking Time:12 Minutes

Ingredients:

- 1-pound collard greens
- 3 bacon strips, chopped
- ¼ cup cherry tomatoes, halved
- 1 tbsp. apple cider vinegar
- 2 tbsp. chicken stock
- Salt and ground black pepper to taste

Directions:

1. Heat a pan over medium heat, add the bacon, stir, and cook until it browns. Add the tomatoes, collard greens, vinegar, stock, salt, and pepper, stir, and cook for 8 minutes.
2. Add more salt, and pepper, stir again gently, divide onto plates, and serve

Nutrition:

Calories 120 ,Fat 8 g ,Carbs 3 g ,Protein 7 g

Sage Salmon Fillet

Servings: 1

Cooking Time: 30 Minutes

Ingredients:

- 4 oz salmon fillet
- ½ teaspoon salt
- 1 teaspoon sesame oil
- ½ teaspoon sage

Directions:

1. Rub the fillet with salt and sage.
2. Place the fish in the tray and sprinkle it with sesame oil.
3. Cook the fish for 25 minutes at 365F.
4. Flip the fish carefully onto another side after 12 minutes of cooking.

Nutrition:

calories 191, fat 11.6, fiber 0.1, carbs 0.2, protein 2

Baked Sweet-potato Fries

Servings:6

Cooking Time: 20 Minutes

Ingredients:

- 1 1/2 teaspoons dried oregano
- 1 teaspoon dried thyme
- 1 teaspoon garlic powder
- 1/2 teaspoon salt
- 2 large sweet potatoes (about 2 pounds), skins on, scrubbed, cut into 1/2-inch thick 4-inch long sticks
- 3 large egg whites (a scant 1/2 cup)
- Vegetable oil, for the parchment
- For the Mediterranean spice:
- Oregano
- Thyme
- Garlic

Directions:

1. Place all of the Mediterranean spice ingredients in a small food processor or a spice grinder; briefly grind or process to blend.
2. Place the oven racks in the middle and upper position; preheat the oven to 450F.
3. Line 2 baking sheets with parchment paper; rub the paper with the oil.
4. Put the potatoes in a microwavable container, cover, and microwave for 2 minutes. Stir gently, cover, and microwave for about 1-2 minutes more or until the pieces are pliable; let rest for about 5 minutes covered. Pour into a platter.
5. In a large-sized bowl, whisk the eggs until frothy. Add the spice mix and whisk again to blend.
6. Working in batches, toss the sweet potatoes in the seasoned egg whites letting the excess liquid drip back into the bowl. Arrange the coated potatoes in a single layer on the preparation ared baking sheets.
7. Bake for 10 minutes; flip the pieces over using a spatula. Rotate the baking sheets from back to front and one to the other; bake for about 15 minutes or until dark golden brown. Serve immediately.

Nutrition:

100 cal., 4 g total fat (0 g sat. fat), 0 mg chol., 60 mg sodium, 230 mg pot., 12 g total carbs., 2 g fiber, 2 g sugar, 3 g protein, 150% vitamin A, 2% vitamin C, 4% calcium, and 6% iron.

Scallions Dip

Servings: 8

Cooking Time: 10 Minutes

Ingredients:

- 6 scallions, chopped
- 1 garlic clove, minced
- 3 tablespoons olive oil
- Salt and black pepper to the taste
- 1 tablespoon lemon juice
- 1 and ½ cups cream cheese, soft
- 2 ounces prosciutto, cooked and crumbled

Directions:

1. In a bowl, mix the scallions with the garlic and the rest of the ingredients except the prosciutto and whisk well.
2. Divide into bowls, sprinkle the prosciutto on top and serve as a party dip.

Nutrition:

calories 144, fat 7.7, fiber 1.4, carbs 6.3, protein 5.5

Blueberry Granola Bars

Servings:3

Cooking Time:10 Minutes

Ingredients:

- ½ C. rolled oats
- 2 tbsp. flaxseeds
- 1 tbsp. sunflower seeds
- 1 tbsp. walnuts, chopped
- 2 tbsp. raisins
- ¾ C. fresh blueberries
- 1 banana, peeled and mashed
- 2 tbsp. dates, pitted and chopped finely
- 1 tbsp. fresh pomegranate juice

Directions:

1. Preheat your oven to 350 degrees F. Lightly, grease an 8-inch baking dish.
2. In a large bowl, add all ingredients and mix until well combined.
3. Place the mixture into preparation ared baking dish evenly and with the back of a spoon, smooth the surface.
4. Bake for about 25 minutes.
5. Remove from oven and keep onto a wire rack to cool.
6. With a sharp knife, cut into desired size bars and serve.

Nutrition:

448 Calories 27g fat 41g carbs 15g protein

Chicken Kale Wraps

Servings: 4

Cooking Time: 10 Minutes

Ingredients:

- 4 kale leaves
- 4 oz chicken fillet
- ½ apple
- 1 tablespoon butter
- ¼ teaspoon chili pepper
- ¾ teaspoon salt
- 1 tablespoon lemon juice
- ¾ teaspoon dried thyme

Directions:

1. Chop the chicken fillet into the small cubes.
2. Then mix up together chicken with chili pepper and salt.
3. Heat up butter in the skillet.
4. Add chicken cubes. Roast them for 4 minutes.
5. Meanwhile, chop the apple into small cubes and add it in the chicken.
6. Mix up well.
7. Sprinkle the ingredients with lemon juice and dried thyme.
8. Cook them for 5 minutes over the medium-high heat.
9. Fill the kale leaves with the hot chicken mixture and wrap

Nutrition:

calories 106, fat 5.1, fiber 1.1, carbs 6.3, protein 9

Vinegar Beet Bites

Servings:4

Cooking Time:30 Minutes

Ingredients:

- 2 beets, sliced
- A pinch of sea salt and black pepper
- 1/3 cup balsamic vinegar
- 1 cup olive oil

Directions:

1. Spread the beet slices on a baking sheet lined with parchment paper, add the rest of the ingredients, toss and bake at 350 degrees F for 30 minutes.
2. Serve the beet bites cold as a snack

Nutrition:

calories 199, fat 5.4, fiber 3.5, carbs 8.5, protein 3.5

Strawberry Frozen Yogurt

Servings: 4

Cooking Time: 15 Minutes

Ingredients:

- 15 ounces of plain yogurt
- 6 ounces of strawberries
- Juice of 1 orange
- 1 tablespoon honey

Directions:

1. Place the strawberries and orange juice into a food processor or blender and blitz until smooth.
2. Press the mixture through a sieve into a large bowl to remove seeds.
3. Stir in the honey and yogurt. Transfer the mixture to an ice-cream maker and follow the manufacturer's instructions.
4. Alternatively, pour the mixture into a container and place in the fridge for 1 hour. Use a fork to whisk it and break up the ice crystals and freeze for 2 hours.

Nutrition:

Calories: 238 ,Sodium: 33 mg ,Dietary Fiber: 1.4 g ,Total Fat: 1.8 g ,Total Carbs: 12.3 g ,Protein: 1.3 g

Tasty Black Bean Dip

Servings: 3

Cooking Time: 18 Minutes

Ingredients:

- 2 cups dry black beans, soaked overnight and drained
- 1 1/2 cups cheese, shredded
- 1 tsp dried oregano
- 1 1/2 tsp chili powder
- 2 cups tomatoes, chopped
- 2 tbsp olive oil
- 1 1/2 tbsp garlic, minced
- 1 medium onion, sliced
- 4 cups vegetable stock
- Pepper
- Salt

Directions:

1. Add all ingredients except cheese into the instant pot.
2. Seal pot with lid and cook on high for 18 minutes.
3. Once done, allow to release pressure naturally. Remove lid. Drain excess water.
4. Add cheese and stir until cheese is melted.
5. Blend bean mixture using an immersion blender until smooth.
6. Serve and enjoy.

Nutrition:

Calories 402 Fat 15.3 g Carbohydrates 46.6 g Sugar 4.4 g Protein 22.2 g Cholesterol 30 mg

Homemade Nutella

Servings:3

Cooking Time:10 Minutes

Ingredients:

- 3/4 cup toasted hazelnuts
- 3 tablespoons peanut oil
- 2 tablespoons cocoa powder
- 3 scoops protein powder
- 1/2 teaspoon vanilla extract
- 2 tablespoons raw honey
- Pinch salt

Directions:

1. Add hazelnuts to your food processor and grind until finely ground; add in peanut oil and process the mixture into butter; add in the remaining ingredients and process until creamy and smooth. Serve with celery or carrot sticks.

Nutrition:

324 Calories 24g fat 20g protein 7g carbs

Oatmeal Cookies

Servings:3

Cooking Time:30 Minutes

Ingredients:

- ¾ C. whole wheat flour
- 1 C. instant oats
- 1½ tsp. organic baking powder
- 1½ tsp. ground cinnamon
- 1/8 tsp. salt
- 1 large organic egg, room temperature
- ½ C. organic honey
- 2 tbsp. coconut oil, melted
- 1 tsp. organic vanilla extract
- 1 C. red apple, cored and chopped finely

Directions:

1. In a large bowl, mix together flour, oats, baking powder, cinnamon and salt.
2. In another bowl, add remaining ingredients except apple and beat until well combined.
3. Add the flour mixture and mix until just combined.
4. Gently, fold in the apple.
5. Refrigerate for about 30 minutes.
6. Preheat the oven to 325 degrees F. Line a large baking sheet with parchment paper.
7. Place about 2 tbsp. of the mixture onto the preparation ared baking sheet in the shape of small mounds.
8. With the back of a spoon, flatten each cookie slightly
9. Bake for about 13-15 minutes.
10. Cool on the pan for 10 minutes before turning out onto a wire rack.
11. Remove from oven and keep onto a wire rack to cool for about 5 minutes.
12. Carefully invert the cookies onto the wire rack to cool completely before serving

Nutrition:

448 Calories 27g fat 41g carbs 15g protein

Chili-lime Cucumber, Jicama, & Apple Sticks

Servings: 3

Cooking Time: 10 Minutes

Ingredients:

- 6 spears cucumber
- 6 spears very ripe apple
- 6 spears jicama (you can use mango instead)
- 1 teaspoon chili lime seasoning
- 2 lime wedges

Directions:

1. In a bowl, mix together cucumber, apple, jicama, lime juice, chili lime seasoning until well combined. Serve garnished with lime wedges. Enjoy!

Nutrition:

324 Calories 24g fat 20g protein 7g carbs

Sardine Meatballs

Servings: 3

Cooking Time: 10 Minutes

Ingredients:

- 11 oz sardines, canned, drained
- 1/3 cup shallot, chopped
- 1 teaspoon chili flakes
- ½ teaspoon salt
- 2 tablespoon wheat flour, whole grain
- 1 egg, beaten
- 1 tablespoon chives, chopped
- 1 teaspoon olive oil
- 1 teaspoon butter

Directions:

1. Put the butter in the skillet and melt it.
2. Add shallot and cook it until translucent.
3. After this, transfer the shallot in the mixing bowl.
4. Add sardines, chili flakes, salt, flour, egg, chives, and mix up until smooth with the help of the fork.
5. Make the medium size cakes and place them in the skillet.
6. Add olive oil.
7. Roast the fish cakes for 3 minutes from each side over the medium heat.
8. Dry the cooked fish cakes with the paper towel if needed and transfer in the serving plates.

Nutrition:

calories 221, fat 12.2, fiber 0.1, carbs 5.4, protein 21.3

Homemade Salsa

Servings: 8

Cooking Time: 30 Minutes

Ingredients:

- 12 oz grape tomatoes, halved
- 1/4 cup fresh cilantro, chopped
- 1 fresh lime juice
- 28 oz tomatoes, crushed
- 1 tbsp garlic, minced
- 1 green bell pepper, chopped
- 1 red bell pepper, chopped
- 2 onions, chopped
- 6 whole tomatoes
- Salt

Directions:

1. Add whole tomatoes into the instant pot and gently smash the tomatoes.
2. Add remaining ingredients except cilantro, lime juice, and salt and stir well.
3. Seal pot with lid and cook on high for 5 minutes.
4. Once done, allow to release pressure naturally for 10 minutes then release remaining using quick release. Remove lid.
5. Add cilantro, lime juice, and salt and stir well.
6. Serve and enjoy.

Nutrition:

Calories 146 Fat 1.2 g Carbohydrates 33.2 g Sugar 4 g Protein 6.9 g Cholesterol 0 mg

Kale Chips

Servings: 3

Cooking Time: 5 Minutes

Ingredients:

- 1 lb. fresh kale leaves, stemmed and torn
- ¼ tsp. cayenne pepper
- Salt, to taste
- 1 tbs. olive oil

Directions:

1. Preheat the oven to 350 degrees F. Line a large baking sheet with a parchment paper.
2. Place the kale pieces onto preparation ared baking sheet in a single layer.
3. Sprinkle the kale with cayenne and salt and drizzle with oil.
4. Bake for about 10-15 minutes.

Nutrition:

242 Calories 25g carbs 12g fat 13g protein

Feta Tomato Sea Bass

Servings:3

Cooking Time:8 Minutes

Ingredients:

- 4 sea bass fillets
- 1 1/2 cups water
- 1 tbsp olive oil
- 1 tsp garlic, minced
- 1 tsp basil, chopped
- 1 tsp parsley, chopped
- 1/2 cup feta cheese, crumbled
- 1 cup can tomatoes, diced
- Pepper
- Salt

Directions:

1. Season fish fillets with pepper and salt.
2. Pour 2 cups of water into the instant pot then place steamer rack in the pot.
3. Place fish fillets on steamer rack in the pot.
4. Seal pot with lid and cook on high for 5 minutes.
5. Once done, release pressure using quick release. Remove lid.
6. Remove fish fillets from the pot and clean the pot.
7. Add oil into the inner pot of instant pot and set the pot on sauté mode.
8. Add garlic and sauté for 1 minute.
9. Add tomatoes, parsley, and basil and stir well and cook for 1 minute.
10. Add fish fillets and top with crumbled cheese and cook for a minute.
11. Serve and enjoy

Nutrition:

Calories 219 Fat 10.1 g Carbohydrates 4 g Sugar 2.8 g Protein 27.1 g Cholesterol 70 mg

Crab Stew

Servings:2

Cooking Time:13 Minutes

Ingredients:

- 1/2 lb lump crab meat
- 2 tbsp heavy cream
- 1 tbsp olive oil
- 2 cups fish stock
- 1/2 lb shrimp, shelled and chopped
- 1 celery stalk, chopped
- 1/2 tsp garlic, chopped
- 1/4 onion, chopped
- Pepper
- Salt

Directions:

1. Add oil into the inner pot of instant pot and set the pot on sauté mode.
2. Add onion and sauté for 3 minutes.
3. Add garlic and sauté for 30 seconds.
4. Add remaining ingredients except for heavy cream and stir well.
5. Seal pot with lid and cook on high for 10 minutes.
6. Once done, release pressure using quick release. Remove lid.
7. Stir in heavy cream and serve

Nutrition:

Calories 376 Fat 25.5 g Carbohydrates 5.8 g Sugar 0.7 g Protein 48.1 g Cholesterol 326 mg

Trail Mix

Servings: 3

Cooking Time: 10 Minutes

Ingredients:

- ¼ cup unsalted roasted peanuts
- ¼ cup whole shelled almonds
- ¼ cup chopped pitted dates
- ¼ cup dried cranberries
- 2 ounces dried apricots

Directions:

1. In a medium bowl, mix together all the ingredients until well combined. Enjoy!

Nutrition:

448 Calories 27g fat 41g carbs 15g protein

Berry & Veggie Gazpacho

Servings: 3

Cooking Time: 30 Minutes

Ingredients:

- 1½ lb. fresh strawberries, hulled and sliced
- ½ C. red bell pepper, seeded and chopped
- 1 small cucumber, peeled, seeded and chopped
- ¼ C. onion, chopped
- ¼ C. fresh basil leaves
- 1 small garlic clove, chopped
- ¼ of small jalapeño pepper, seeded and chopped
- 1 tbsp. olive oil
- 3 tbsp. balsamic vinegar

Directions:

1. In a high-speed blender, add all ingredients and pulse until smooth.
2. Transfer the gazpacho into a large bowl.
3. Cover and refrigerate to chill completely before serving.

Nutrition:

448 Calories 27g fat 41g carbs 15g protein

Meat-filled Phyllo (samboosek)

Servings:1

Cooking Time:10 Minutes

Ingredients:

- 1 lb. ground beef or lamb
- 1 medium yellow onion, finely chopped
- 1 TB. seven spices
- 1 tsp. salt
- 1 pkg. frozen phyllo dough (12 sheets)
- 2/3 cup butter, melted

Directions:

1. In a medium skillet over medium heat, brown beef for 3 minutes, breaking up chunks with a wooden spoon.
2. Add yellow onion, seven spices, and salt, and cook for 5 to 7 minutes or until beef is browned and onions are translucent. Set aside, and let cool.
3. Place first sheet of phyllo on your work surface, brush with melted butter, lay second sheet of phyllo on top, and brush with melted butter. Cut sheets into 3-inch-wide strips.
4. Spoon 2 tablespoons meat filling at end of each strip, and fold end strip to cover meat and form a triangle. Fold pointed end up and over to the opposite end, and you should see a triangle forming. Continue to fold up and then over until you come to the end of strip.
5. Place phyllo pies on a baking sheet, seal side down, and brush tops with butter. Repeat with remaining phyllo and filling.
6. Bake for 10 minutes or until golden brown.
7. Remove from the oven and set aside for 5 minutes before serving warm or at room temperature

Nutrition:

242 Calories 25g carbs 12g fat 13g protein

Raw Turmeric Cashew Nut & Coconut Balls

Servings:3

Cooking Time:10 Minutes

Ingredients:

- 1 cup raw cashews
- 1 1/2 cup shredded coconut
- 1 tablespoon raw honey
- 3 teaspoons ground turmeric
- 1 teaspoon cinnamon
- 1 teaspoon ground ginger
- 1 teaspoon black pepper
- 1/2 teaspoon sea salt

Directions:

1. In a food processor, process coconut until almost oily; add in the rest of the ingredients and process until cashews are finely chopped.
2. Press the mixture into bite-sized balls and arrange them on a baking tray. Refrigerate until firm before serving

Nutrition:

324 Calories 24g fat 20g protein 7g carbs

Ginger Tahini Dip With Veggies

Servings: 3

Cooking Time: 10 Minutes

Ingredients:

- ½ cup tahini
- 1 teaspoon grated garlic
- 2 teaspoons ground turmeric
- 1 tablespoon grated fresh ginger
- ¼ cup apple cider vinegar
- ¼ cup water
- ½ teaspoon salt

Directions:

1. In a bowl, whisk together tahini, turmeric, ginger, water, vinegar, garlic, and salt until well blended. Serve with assorted veggies

Nutrition:

448 Calories 27g fat 41g carbs 15g protein

Crunchy Veggie Chips

Servings:3

Cooking Time:17 Minutes

Ingredients:

- 1 cup thinly sliced portobello mushrooms
- 1 cup thinly sliced zucchini
- 1 cup thinly sliced sweet potatoes
- 1 tablespoon extra-virgin olive oil
- Pinch of sea salt
- Pinch of pepper

Directions:

1. Place veggies in a baking dish and drizzle with olive oil; sprinkle with salt and pepper and toss to coat well; bake at 325°F for about 12 minutes or until crunchy. Enjoy!

Nutrition:

448 Calories 27g fat 41g carbs 15g protein

Honey Garlic Shrimp

Servings:3

Cooking Time:5 Minutes

Ingredients:

- 1 lb shrimp, peeled and deveined
- 1/4 cup honey
- 1 tbsp garlic, minced
- 1 tbsp ginger, minced
- 1 tbsp olive oil
- 1/4 cup fish stock
- Pepper
- Salt

Directions:

1. Add shrimp into the large bowl. Add remaining ingredients over shrimp and toss well.
2. Transfer shrimp into the instant pot and stir well.
3. Seal pot with lid and cook on high for 5 minutes.
4. Once done, release pressure using quick release. Remove lid.
5. Serve and enjoy.

Nutrition:

Calories 240 Fat 5.6 g Carbohydrates 20.9 g Sugar 17.5 g Protein 26.5 g Cholesterol 239 mg

Pita Chips

Servings:3

Cooking Time:30 Minutes

Ingredients:

- 6 whole wheat pitas, cut each into 8 wedges
- 2 tsp. olive oil
- Red chili powder, to taste
- Garlic powder, to taste
- Pinch of salt

Directions:

1. Preheat the oven to 400 degrees F.
2. In the bottom of a large baking sheet, place the pita wedges.
3. Brush the both sides of each with oil and sprinkle with chili powder, garlic powder and salt.
4. Now, arrange the pita wedges in a single layer.
5. Bake for about 8 minutes or until golden brown.
6. Serve with your favorite dip

Nutrition:

242 Calories 25g carbs 12g fat 13g protein

Leeks And Calamari Mix

Servings:6

Cooking Time:15 Minutes

Ingredients:

- 2 tablespoon avocado oil
- 2 leeks, chopped
- 1 red onion, chopped
- Salt and black to the taste
- 1 pound calamari rings
- 1 tablespoon parsley, chopped
- 1 tablespoon chives, chopped
- 2 tablespoons tomato paste

Directions:

1. Heat up a pan with the avocado oil over medium heat, add the leeks and the onion, stir and sauté for 5 minutes.
2. Add the rest of the ingredients, toss, simmer over medium heat for 10 minutes, divide into bowls and serve

Nutrition:

calories 238, fat 9, fiber 5.6, carbs 14.4, protein 8.4

Cucumber Rolls

Servings: 3

Cooking Time: 10 Minutes

Ingredients:

- 1 big cucumber, sliced lengthwise
- 1 tablespoon parsley, chopped
- 8 ounces canned tuna, drained and mashed
- Salt and black pepper to the taste
- 1 teaspoon lime juice

Directions:

1. Arrange cucumber slices on a working surface, divide the rest of the ingredients, and roll.
2. Arrange all the rolls on a platter and serve as an appetizer.

Nutrition:

calories 200, fat 6, fiber 3.4, carbs 7.6, protein 3.5

Parmesan Chips

Servings: 4

Cooking Time: 20 Minutes

Ingredients:

- 1 zucchini
- 2 oz Parmesan, grated
- ½ teaspoon paprika
- 1 teaspoon olive oil

Directions:

1. Trim zucchini and slice it into the chips with the help of the vegetable slices.
2. Then mix up together Parmesan and paprika.
3. Sprinkle the zucchini chips with olive oil.
4. After this, dip every zucchini slice in the cheese mixture.
5. Place the zucchini chips in the lined baking tray and bake for 20 minutes at 375F.
6. Flip the zucchini sliced onto another side after 10 minutes of cooking.
7. Chill the cooked chips well.

Nutrition:

calories 64, fat 4.3, fiber 0.6, carbs 2.3, protein 5.2

Grape, Celery & Parsley Reviver

Servings: 2

Cooking Time: 10 Minutes

Ingredients:

- 75g 3ozred grapes
- 3 sticks of celery
- 1 avocado, de-stoned and peeled
- 1 tablespoon fresh parsley
- ½ teaspoon matcha powder

Directions:

1. Place all of the ingredients into a blender with enough water to cover them and blitz until smooth and creamy. Add crushed ice to make it even more refreshing.

Nutrition:

Calories 334, Fat 1.5 g, Carbohydrate 42.9 g, Protein 6 g

Tomato Triangles

Servings: 6

Cooking Time: 10 Minutes

Ingredients:

- 6 corn tortillas
- 1 tablespoon cream cheese
- 1 tablespoon ricotta cheese
- ½ teaspoon minced garlic
- 1 tablespoon fresh dill, chopped
- 2 tomatoes, sliced

Directions:

1. Cut every tortilla into 2 triangles.
2. Then mix up together cream cheese, ricotta cheese, minced garlic, and dill.
3. Spread 6 triangles with cream cheese mixture.
4. Then place sliced tomato on them and cover with remaining tortilla triangles.

Nutrition:

calories 71, fat 1.6, fiber 2.1, carbs 12.8, protein 2.3

Asparagus Frittata

Servings: 4

Cooking Time: 15 Minutes

Ingredients:

- ¼ cup onion, chopped
- Drizzle of olive oil
- 1-pound asparagus spears, cut into 1-inch pieces
- Salt and ground black pepper to taste
- 4 eggs, whisked
- 1 cup cheddar cheese, grated

Directions:

1. Heat a pan with the oil over medium-high heat, add the onions, stir, and cook for 3 minutes. Add the asparagus, stir, and cook for 6 minutes. Add the eggs, stir, and cook for 3 minutes.
2. Add the salt and pepper sprinkle with the cheese, put in an oven, and broil for 3 minutes.
3. Divide the frittata onto plates and serve.

Nutrition:

Calories 200 ,Fat 12 g ,Carbs 5 g ,Protein 14 g

Salmon And Broccoli

Servings: 3

Cooking Time: 20 Minutes

Ingredients:

- 2 tablespoons balsamic vinegar
- 1 broccoli head, florets separated
- 4 pieces salmon fillets, skinless
- 1 big red onion, roughly chopped
- 1 tablespoon olive oil
- Sea salt and black pepper to the taste

Directions:

1. In a baking dish, combine the salmon with the broccoli and the rest of the ingredients, introduce in the oven and bake at 390 degrees F for 20 minutes.
2. Divide the mix between plates and serve.

Nutrition:

calories 302, fat 15.5, fiber 8.5, carbs 18.9, protein 19.8

Chili Mango And Watermelon Salsa

Servings: 8

Cooking Time: 10 Minutes

Ingredients:

- 1 red tomato, chopped
- Salt and black pepper to the taste
- 1 cup watermelon, seedless, peeled and cubed
- 1 red onion, chopped
- 2 mangos, peeled and chopped
- 2 chili peppers, chopped
- ¼ cup cilantro, chopped
- 3 tablespoons lime juice
- Pita chips for serving

Directions:

1. In a bowl, mix the tomato with the watermelon, the onion and the rest of the ingredients except the pita chips and toss well.
2. Divide the mix into small cups and serve with pita chips on the side.

Nutrition:

calories 62, fat 4.7, fiber 1.3, carbs 3.9, protein 2.3

Chia Crackers

Servings: 24

Cooking Time:

Ingredients:

- 1/2 cup pecans, chopped
- 1/2 cup chia seeds
- 1/2 tsp. cayenne pepper
- 1 cup water
- 1/4 cup nutritional yeast
- 1/2 cup pumpkin seeds
- 1/4 cup ground flax
- Salt and pepper, to taste

Directions:

1. Mix around 1/2 cup of chia seeds and 1 cup of water. Keep it aside.
2. Take another bowl and combine all the remaining ingredients. Combine well and stir in the chia water mixture until you obtained dough.
3. Transfer the dough onto a baking sheet and roll it out into a ¼"-thick dough.
4. Transfer into a preheated oven at 325°F and bake for about ½ hour.
5. Take out from the oven, flip over the dough, and cut it into desired cracker shaped-squares.
6. Spread and back again for a further half an hour, or until crispy and browned.
7. Once done, take them out from the oven and let them cool at room temperature. Enjoy!

Nutrition:

Calories: 41 ,Fats: 3.1 g ,Carbs: 2 g ,Protein: 2 g

Lavash Roll Ups

Servings:4

Cooking Time:10 Minutes

Ingredients:

- 2 lavash wraps (whole-wheat)
- 1/4 cup roasted red peppers, sliced
- 1/4 cup black olives, sliced
- 1/2 cup hummus of choice
- 1/2 cup grape tomatoes, halved
- 1 Medium cucumber, sliced
- Fresh dill, for garnish

Directions:

1. Lay out the lavash wraps on a clean surface. Evenly spread hummus over each piece.
2. Layer the cucumbers across the wraps, about 1/2-inch from each other, leaving about 2-icnh empty space at the bottom of the wrap for rolling purposes.
3. Place the roasted pepper slices around the cucumbers. Sprinkle with black olives and the tomatoes. Garnish with freshly chopped dill.
4. Tightly roll each wrap, using the hummus at the end to almost glue the wrap into a roll.
5. Slice each roll into 4 equal pieces. Secure each piece by sticking a toothpick through the center of each roll slice.
6. Lay each on a serving bowl or tray; garnish more with fresh dill.

Nutrition:

250 cal, 8 g total fat (0.5 g sat. fat), 0 mg chol., 440 mg sodium, 340 mg pot., 43 total carbs., 40 g fiber, 3 g sugar, 10 g protein, 15% vitamin A, 25% vitamin C, 6% calcium, and 8% iron.

Pepper Salmon Skewers

Servings:5

Cooking Time:15 Minutes

Ingredients:

- 1.5-pound salmon fillet
- ½ cup Plain yogurt
- 1 teaspoon paprika
- 1 teaspoon turmeric
- 1 teaspoon red pepper
- 1 teaspoon salt
- 1 teaspoon dried cilantro
- 1 teaspoon sunflower oil
- ½ teaspoon ground nutmeg

Directions:

1. For the marinade: mix up together Plain yogurt, paprika, turmeric red pepper, salt, and ground nutmeg.
2. Chop the salmon fillet roughly and put it in the yogurt mixture.
3. Mix up well and marinate for 25 minutes.
4. Then skew the fish on the skewers.
5. Sprinkle the skewers with sunflower oil and place in the tray.
6. Bake the salmon skewers for 15 minutes at 375F.

Nutrition:

calories 217, fat 9.9, fiber 0.6, carbs 4.2, protein 28.1

Garlic Mussels

Servings: 4

Cooking Time: 10 Minutes

Ingredients:

- 1-pound mussels
- 1 chili pepper, chopped
- 1 cup chicken stock
- ½ cup milk
- 1 teaspoon olive oil
- 1 teaspoon minced garlic
- 1 teaspoon ground coriander
- ½ teaspoon salt
- 1 cup fresh parsley, chopped
- 4 tablespoons lemon juice

Directions:

1. Pour milk in the saucepan.
2. Add chili pepper, chicken stock, olive oil, minced garlic, ground coriander, salt, and lemon juice.
3. Bring the liquid to boil and add mussels.
4. Boil the mussel for 4 minutes or until they will open shells.
5. Then add chopped parsley and mix up the meal well.
6. Remove it from the heat

Nutrition:

calories 136, fat 4.7, fiber 0.6, carbs 7.5, protein 15.3

Superfood Spiced Apricot-sesame Bliss Balls

Servings:3

Cooking Time:30 Minutes

Ingredients:

- 2 tablespoons sesame seeds
- 1 cup apricots
- 1 cup natural gluten-free muesli
- 1 cup almonds
- 2 tablespoons raw honey
- 1 teaspoon ground cinnamon

Directions:

- In a food processor, process almonds until finely chopped; add in raw honey, muesli, apricots, and cinnamon and process until very smooth.
- Add sesame seeds in a shallow dish. Roll two tablespoons of the almond mixture into bite-sized balls and then roll them into the sesame seeds until well coated.
- Arrange them on a tray and refrigerate until set. Serve and store the rest in an airtight container.

Nutrition:

448 Calories 27g fat 41g carbs 15g protein

Halibut And Quinoa Mix

Servings: 4

Cooking Time: 30 Minutes

Ingredients:

- 4 halibut fillets, boneless
- 2 tablespoons olive oil
- 1 teaspoon rosemary, dried
- 2 teaspoons cumin, ground
- 1 tablespoons coriander, ground
- 2 teaspoons cinnamon powder
- 2 teaspoons oregano, dried
- A pinch of salt and black pepper
- 2 cups quinoa, cooked
- 1 cup cherry tomatoes, halved
- 1 avocado, peeled, pitted and sliced
- 1 cucumber, cubed
- ½ cup black olives, pitted and sliced
- Juice of 1 lemon

Directions:

- In a bowl, combine the fish with the rosemary, cumin, coriander, cinnamon, oregano, salt and pepper and toss.
- Heat up a pan with the oil over medium heat, add the fish, and sear for 2 minutes on each side.
- Introduce the pan in the oven and bake the fish at 425 degrees F for 7 minutes.
- Meanwhile, in a bowl, mix the quinoa with the remaining ingredients, toss and divide between plates.
- Add the fish next to the quinoa mix and serve right away.

Nutrition:

calories 364, fat 15.4, fiber 11.2, carbs 56.4, protein 24.5

Orange-spiced Pumpkin Hummus

Servings:4

Cooking Time:5 Minutes

Ingredients:

- 1 tbsp. maple syrup
- 1/2 tsp. salt
- 1 can (16 oz.) garbanzo beans
- 1/8 tsp. ginger or nutmeg
- 1 cup canned pumpkin Blend,
- 1/8 tsp. cinnamon
- 1/4 cup tahini
- 1 tbsp. fresh orange juice
- Pinch of orange zest, for garnish
- 1 tbsp. apple cider vinegar

Directions:

- Mix all the ingredients in a food processor or blender until slightly chunky.
- Serve right away, and enjoy!

Nutrition:

Calories: 291 ,Fats: 22.9 g ,Carbs: 15 g ,Protein: 12 g

Artichoke Skewers

Servings: 4

Cooking Time: 10 Minutes

Ingredients:

- 4 prosciutto slices
- 4 artichoke hearts, canned
- 4 kalamata olives
- 4 cherry tomatoes
- ¼ teaspoon cayenne pepper
- ¼ teaspoon sunflower oil

Directions:

- Skewer prosciutto slices, artichoke hearts, kalamata olives, and cherry tomatoes on the wooden skewers.
- Sprinkle antipasto skewers with sunflower oil and cayenne pepper.

Nutrition:

calories 152, fat 3.7, fiber 10.8, carbs 23.2, protein 11.1

Honey Balsamic Salmon

Servings: 2

Cooking Time: 3 Minutes

Ingredients:

- 2 salmon fillets
- 1/4 tsp red pepper flakes
- 2 tbsp honey
- 2 tbsp balsamic vinegar
- 1 cup of water
- Pepper
- Salt

Directions:

- Pour water into the instant pot and place trivet in the pot.
- In a small bowl, mix together honey, red pepper flakes, and vinegar.
- Brush fish fillets with honey mixture and place on top of the trivet.
- Seal pot with lid and cook on high for 3 minutes.
- Once done, release pressure using quick release. Remove lid.
- Serve and enjoy.

Nutrition:

Calories 303 Fat 11 g Carbohydrates 17.6 g Sugar 17.3 g Protein 34.6 g Cholesterol 78 mg

Conclusion

Eating can improve and alleviate symptoms of liver cirrhosis. It is important to stay hydrated with water, juice or other fluids because dehydration will cause a build up of toxins in the body. A diet low in fat but high in protein and carbohydrates help maintain proper weight while giving essential nutrients for fighting off infection. The list goes on! But one thing that you need to know about your liver is that it's still working hard even if you have lost 80% function due to alcohol abuse.

Cirrhosis is an irreversible, chronic liver disease that can lead to complete organ failure. The cirrhosis diet plays a major role in the course of this condition and there are both eating tips for people with liver cirrhosis as well as information on how the functions of the liver work. You're not alone; many people suffer from this disease without knowing they are living with it until later stages when the risks increase considerably, so let's take care of our livers so we can live better!